Goals

Carbs: _____________   Fats: _____________   Proteins: _____________

Weight: _____________   Waist: _____________   Hips: _____________   Thighs:

Arms: _____________   Other: _____________

Cheat Meal

What Day? _____________________________

What Meal? _____________________________

What Food? _____________________________

Make your cheat meal something indulgent, but still keto-friendly to stay on track! i.e. Keto Ice cream, brownies, etc.

Meal Ideas

<table>
<tr><td>MONDAY</td><td>Macros: _____carbs _____fats _____proteins</td></tr>
<tr><td>TUESDAY</td><td>Macros: _____carbs _____fats _____proteins</td></tr>
<tr><td>WEDNESDAY</td><td>Macros: _____carbs _____fats _____proteins</td></tr>
<tr><td>THURSDAY</td><td>Macros: _____carbs _____fats _____proteins</td></tr>
<tr><td>FRIDAY</td><td>Macros: _____carbs _____fats _____proteins</td></tr>
<tr><td>SATURDAY</td><td>Macros: _____carbs _____fats _____proteins</td></tr>
<tr><td>SUNDAY</td><td>Macros: _____carbs _____fats _____proteins</td></tr>
</table>

End of Week Stats

Carbs: __________   Fats: __________   Proteins: __________

Weight: __________   Waist: __________   Hips: __________   Thighs: __________

Arms: __________   Other: __________

Take Inventory

Rate these items on a scale of 1-5, 1 being worst, 5 being best. Add your own if you wish.

Sleep __________   __________   __________

Energy __________   __________   __________

Satiety __________   __________   __________

Mental Clarity __________   __________   __________

Notes

____

____

____

____

____

____

____

____

____

____

Notes

Goals

Carbs: __________   Fats: __________   Proteins: __________

Weight: __________   Waist: __________   Hips: __________   Thighs: __________

Arms: __________   Other: __________

Cheat Meal

What Day? __________________________

What Meal? __________________________

What Food? __________________________

Make your cheat meal something indulgent, but still keto-friendly to stay on track! i.e. Keto Ice cream, brownies, etc.

Meal Ideas

____

____

____

____

____

____

____

____

____

____

____

MONDAY

Macros: _____carbs _____fats _____proteins

TUESDAY

Macros: _____carbs _____fats _____proteins

WEDNESDAY

Macros: _____carbs _____fats _____proteins

THURSDAY

Macros: _____carbs _____fats _____proteins

FRIDAY

Macros: _____carbs _____fats _____proteins

SATURDAY

Macros: _____carbs _____fats _____proteins

SUNDAY

Macros: _____carbs _____fats _____proteins

End of Week Stats

Carbs: __________   Fats: __________   Proteins: __________

Weight: __________   Waist: __________   Hips: __________   Thighs: __________

Arms: __________   Other: __________

Take Inventory

Rate these items on a scale of 1-5, 1 being worst, 5 being best. Add your own if you wish.

Sleep __________   __________   __________

Energy __________   __________   __________

Satiety __________   __________   __________

Mental Clarity __________   __________   __________

Notes

____

____

____

____

____

____

____

____

____

____

____

____

Notes

Goals

Carbs: ___________   Fats: ___________   Proteins: ___________

Weight: ___________   Waist: ___________   Hips: ___________   Thighs: ___________

Arms: ___________   Other: ___________

Cheat Meal

What Day? _______________________

What Meal? _______________________

What Food? _______________________

Make your cheat meal something indulgent, but still keto-friendly to stay on track! i.e. Keto Ice cream, brownies, etc.

Meal Ideas

____

____

____

____

____

____

____

____

____

____

____

____

MONDAY	
	Macros: _____carbs _____fats _____proteins
TUESDAY	
	Macros: _____carbs _____fats _____proteins
WEDNESDAY	
	Macros: _____carbs _____fats _____proteins
THURSDAY	
	Macros: _____carbs _____fats _____proteins
FRIDAY	
	Macros: _____carbs _____fats _____proteins
SATURDAY	
	Macros: _____carbs _____fats _____proteins
SUNDAY	
	Macros: _____carbs _____fats _____proteins

End of Week Stats

Carbs: _________   Fats: _________   Proteins: _________

Weight: _________   Waist: _________   Hips: _________   Thighs: _________

Arms: _________   Other: _________

Take Inventory

Rate these items on a scale of 1-5, 1 being worst, 5 being best. Add your own if you wish.

Sleep   _________   _________________________   _________

Energy   _________   _________________________   _________

Satiety   _________   _________________________   _________

Mental Clarity   _________   _________________________   _________

Notes

____

____

____

____

____

____

____

____

____

____

____

____

Notes

Goals

Carbs: __________   Fats: __________   Proteins: __________

Weight: __________   Waist: __________   Hips: __________   Thighs: __________

Arms: __________   Other: __________

Cheat Meal

What Day?   __________________________

What Meal?   __________________________

What Food?   __________________________

Make your cheat meal something indulgent, but still keto-friendly to stay on track! i.e. Keto Ice cream, brownies, etc.

Meal Ideas

____

____

____

____

____

____

____

____

____

____

____

MONDAY

Macros: _____carbs _____fats _____proteins

TUESDAY

Macros: _____carbs _____fats _____proteins

WEDNESDAY

Macros: _____carbs _____fats _____proteins

THURSDAY

Macros: _____carbs _____fats _____proteins

FRIDAY

Macros: _____carbs _____fats _____proteins

SATURDAY

Macros: _____carbs _____fats _____proteins

SUNDAY

Macros: _____carbs _____fats _____proteins

End of Week Stats

Carbs: _________   Fats: _________   Proteins: _________

Weight: ________   Waist: ________   Hips: ________   Thighs: ________

Arms: ________   Other: ________

Take Inventory

Rate these items on a scale of 1-5, 1 being worst, 5 being best. Add your own if you wish.

Sleep _________   _____________________   _________

Energy _________   _____________________   _________

Satiety _________   _____________________   _________

Mental Clarity _________   _____________________   _________

Notes

____

____

____

____

____

____

____

____

____

____

____

Notes

Goals

Carbs: _________   Fats: _________   Proteins: _________

Weight: _________   Waist: _________   Hips: _________   Thighs: _________

Arms: _________   Other: _________

Cheat Meal

What Day?   _______________________

What Meal?   _______________________

What Food?   _______________________

Make your cheat meal something indulgent, but still keto-friendly to stay on track! i.e. Keto Ice cream, brownies, etc.

Meal Ideas

____

____

____

____

____

____

____

____

____

____

Day	
MONDAY	Macros: _____carbs _____fats _____proteins
TUESDAY	Macros: _____carbs _____fats _____proteins
WEDNESDAY	Macros: _____carbs _____fats _____proteins
THURSDAY	Macros: _____carbs _____fats _____proteins
FRIDAY	Macros: _____carbs _____fats _____proteins
SATURDAY	Macros: _____carbs _____fats _____proteins
SUNDAY	Macros: _____carbs _____fats _____proteins

End of Week Stats

Carbs: _________   Fats: _________   Proteins: _________

Weight: _________   Waist: _________   Hips: _________   Thighs: _________

Arms: _________   Other: _________

Take Inventory

Rate these items on a scale of 1-5, 1 being worst, 5 being best. Add your own if you wish.

Sleep   _________   _________________   _________

Energy   _________   _________________   _________

Satiety   _________   _________________   _________

Mental Clarity   _________   _________________   _________

Notes

____

____

____

____

____

____

____

____

____

____

____

Notes

Goals

Carbs: _________   Fats: _________   Proteins: _________

Weight: _________   Waist: _________   Hips: _________   Thighs: _________

Arms: _________   Other: _________

Cheat Meal

What Day? _________________________

What Meal? _________________________

What Food? _________________________

Make your cheat meal something indulgent, but still keto-friendly to stay on track! i.e. Keto Ice cream, brownies, etc.

Meal Ideas

____

____

____

____

____

____

____

____

____

____

____

MONDAY

Macros: _____carbs _____fats _____proteins

TUESDAY

Macros: _____carbs _____fats _____proteins

WEDNESDAY

Macros: _____carbs _____fats _____proteins

THURSDAY

Macros: _____carbs _____fats _____proteins

FRIDAY

Macros: _____carbs _____fats _____proteins

SATURDAY

Macros: _____carbs _____fats _____proteins

SUNDAY

Macros: _____carbs _____fats _____proteins

End of Week Stats

Carbs: __________   Fats: __________   Proteins: __________

Weight: __________   Waist: __________   Hips: __________   Thighs: __________

Arms: __________   Other: __________

Take Inventory

Rate these items on a scale of 1-5, 1 being worst, 5 being best. Add your own if you wish.

Sleep __________   __________   __________

Energy __________   __________   __________

Satiety __________   __________   __________

Mental Clarity __________   __________   __________

Notes

____

____

____

____

____

____

____

____

____

____

____

____

Notes

Goals

Carbs: _________   Fats: _________   Proteins: _________

Weight: _________   Waist: _________   Hips: _________   Thighs: _________

Arms: _________   Other: _________

Cheat Meal

What Day? _______________________

What Meal? _______________________

What Food? _______________________

Make your cheat meal something indulgent, but still keto-friendly to stay on track! i.e. Keto Ice cream, brownies, etc.

Meal Ideas

____

____

____

____

____

____

____

____

____

____

____

____

MONDAY	
	Macros: _____carbs _____fats _____proteins

TUESDAY	
	Macros: _____carbs _____fats _____proteins

WEDNESDAY	
	Macros: _____carbs _____fats _____proteins

THURSDAY	
	Macros: _____carbs _____fats _____proteins

FRIDAY	
	Macros: _____carbs _____fats _____proteins

SATURDAY	
	Macros: _____carbs _____fats _____proteins

SUNDAY	
	Macros: _____carbs _____fats _____proteins

End of Week Stats

Carbs: __________   Fats: __________   Proteins: __________

Weight: __________   Waist: __________   Hips: __________   Thighs: __________

Arms: __________   Other: __________

Take Inventory

Rate these items on a scale of 1-5, 1 being worst, 5 being best. Add your own if you wish.

Sleep __________   __________________   __________

Energy __________   __________________   __________

Satiety __________   __________________   __________

Mental Clarity __________   __________________   __________

Notes

____

____

____

____

____

____

____

____

____

____

____

Notes

Goals

Carbs: __________   Fats: __________   Proteins: __________

Weight: __________   Waist: __________   Hips: __________   Thighs: __________

Arms: __________   Other: __________

Cheat Meal

What Day? __________________________

What Meal? __________________________

What Food? __________________________

Make your cheat meal something indulgent, but still keto-friendly to stay on track! i.e. Keto Ice cream, brownies, etc.

Meal Ideas

____

____

____

____

____

____

____

____

____

____

<table>
<tr><td>MONDAY</td><td>Macros: _ _ _ _ _carbs _ _ _ _ _fats _ _ _ _ _proteins</td></tr>
<tr><td>TUESDAY</td><td>Macros: _ _ _ _ _carbs _ _ _ _ _fats _ _ _ _ _proteins</td></tr>
<tr><td>WEDNESDAY</td><td>Macros: _ _ _ _ _carbs _ _ _ _ _fats _ _ _ _ _proteins</td></tr>
<tr><td>THURSDAY</td><td>Macros: _ _ _ _ _carbs _ _ _ _ _fats _ _ _ _ _proteins</td></tr>
<tr><td>FRIDAY</td><td>Macros: _ _ _ _ _carbs _ _ _ _ _fats _ _ _ _ _proteins</td></tr>
<tr><td>SATURDAY</td><td>Macros: _ _ _ _ _carbs _ _ _ _ _fats _ _ _ _ _proteins</td></tr>
<tr><td>SUNDAY</td><td>Macros: _ _ _ _ _carbs _ _ _ _ _fats _ _ _ _ _proteins</td></tr>
</table>

End of Week Stats

Carbs: __________   Fats: __________   Proteins: __________

Weight: __________   Waist: __________   Hips: __________   Thighs: __________

Arms: __________   Other: __________

Take Inventory

Rate these items on a scale of 1–5, 1 being worst, 5 being best. Add your own if you wish.

Sleep   __________

Energy   __________

Satiety   __________

Mental Clarity __________

Notes

____

____

____

____

____

____

____

____

____

____

____

____

Notes

Goals

Carbs: __________   Fats: __________   Proteins: __________

Weight: __________   Waist: __________   Hips: __________   Thighs: __________

Arms: __________   Other: __________

Cheat Meal

What Day? ______________________

What Meal? ______________________

What Food? ______________________

Make your cheat meal something indulgent, but still keto-friendly to stay on track! i.e. Keto Ice cream, brownies, etc.

Meal Ideas

____

____

____

____

____

____

____

____

____

____

____

MONDAY

Macros: _____carbs _____fats _____proteins

TUESDAY

Macros: _____carbs _____fats _____proteins

WEDNESDAY

Macros: _____carbs _____fats _____proteins

THURSDAY

Macros: _____carbs _____fats _____proteins

FRIDAY

Macros: _____carbs _____fats _____proteins

SATURDAY

Macros: _____carbs _____fats _____proteins

SUNDAY

Macros: _____carbs _____fats _____proteins

End of Week Stats

Carbs: __________   Fats: __________   Proteins: __________

Weight: __________   Waist: __________   Hips: __________   Thighs: __________

Arms: __________   Other: __________

Take Inventory

Rate these items on a scale of 1-5, 1 being worst, 5 being best. Add your own if you wish.

Sleep __________

Energy __________

Satiety __________

Mental Clarity __________

Notes

____

____

____

____

____

____

____

____

____

____

____

____

Notes

Goals

Carbs: __________   Fats: __________   Proteins: __________

Weight: __________   Waist: __________   Hips: __________   Thighs: __________

Arms: __________   Other: __________

Cheat Meal

What Day? _______________________

What Meal? _______________________

What Food? _______________________

Make your cheat meal something indulgent, but still keto-friendly to stay on track! i.e. Keto Ice cream, brownies, etc.

Meal Ideas

____

____

____

____

____

____

____

____

____

____

____

____

<table>
<tr><td>MONDAY</td><td>Macros: _ _ _ _ _carbs _ _ _ _ _fats _ _ _ _ _proteins</td></tr>
<tr><td>TUESDAY</td><td>Macros: _ _ _ _ _carbs _ _ _ _ _fats _ _ _ _ _proteins</td></tr>
<tr><td>WEDNESDAY</td><td>Macros: _ _ _ _ _carbs _ _ _ _ _fats _ _ _ _ _proteins</td></tr>
<tr><td>THURSDAY</td><td>Macros: _ _ _ _ _carbs _ _ _ _ _fats _ _ _ _ _proteins</td></tr>
<tr><td>FRIDAY</td><td>Macros: _ _ _ _ _carbs _ _ _ _ _fats _ _ _ _ _proteins</td></tr>
<tr><td>SATURDAY</td><td>Macros: _ _ _ _ _carbs _ _ _ _ _fats _ _ _ _ _proteins</td></tr>
<tr><td>SUNDAY</td><td>Macros: _ _ _ _ _carbs _ _ _ _ _fats _ _ _ _ _proteins</td></tr>
</table>

End of Week Stats

Carbs: _________   Fats: _________   Proteins: _________

Weight: _________   Waist: _________   Hips: _________   Thighs: _________

Arms: _________   Other: _________

Take Inventory

Rate these items on a scale of 1-5, 1 being worst, 5 being best. Add your own if you wish.

Sleep _________   _________________   _________

Energy _________   _________________   _________

Satiety _________   _________________   _________

Mental Clarity _________   _________________   _________

Notes

____

____

____

____

____

____

____

____

____

____

____

Notes

Notes

Goals

Carbs: __________   Fats: __________   Proteins: __________

Weight: __________   Waist: __________   Hips: __________   Thighs: __________

Arms: __________   Other: __________

Cheat Meal

What Day? _______________________

What Meal? _______________________

What Food? _______________________

Make your cheat meal something indulgent, but still keto-friendly to stay on track! i.e. Keto Ice cream, brownies, etc.

Meal Ideas

____

____

____

____

____

____

____

____

____

____

____

MONDAY	
	Macros: _____carbs _____fats _____proteins
TUESDAY	
	Macros: _____carbs _____fats _____proteins
WEDNESDAY	
	Macros: _____carbs _____fats _____proteins
THURSDAY	
	Macros: _____carbs _____fats _____proteins
FRIDAY	
	Macros: _____carbs _____fats _____proteins
SATURDAY	
	Macros: _____carbs _____fats _____proteins
SUNDAY	
	Macros: _____carbs _____fats _____proteins

End of Week Stats

Carbs: __________   Fats: __________   Proteins: __________

Weight: __________   Waist: __________   Hips: __________   Thighs: __________

Arms: __________   Other: __________

Take Inventory

Rate these items on a scale of 1-5, 1 being worst, 5 being best. Add your own if you wish.

Sleep __________   __________________   __________

Energy __________   __________________   __________

Satiety __________   __________________   __________

Mental Clarity __________   __________________   __________

Notes

____

____

____

____

____

____

____

____

____

____

____

Notes

Goals

Carbs: __________   Fats: __________   Proteins: __________

Weight: __________   Waist: __________   Hips: __________   Thighs: __________

Arms: __________   Other: __________

Cheat Meal

What Day? __________________________

What Meal? __________________________

What Food? __________________________

Make your cheat meal something indulgent, but still keto-friendly to stay on track! i.e. Keto Ice cream, brownies, etc.

Meal Ideas

____

____

____

____

____

____

____

____

____

____

____

MONDAY

Macros: _ _ _ _ _carbs _ _ _ _ _fats _ _ _ _ _proteins

TUESDAY

Macros: _ _ _ _ _carbs _ _ _ _ _fats _ _ _ _ _proteins

WEDNESDAY

Macros: _ _ _ _ _carbs _ _ _ _ _fats _ _ _ _ _proteins

THURSDAY

Macros: _ _ _ _ _carbs _ _ _ _ _fats _ _ _ _ _proteins

FRIDAY

Macros: _ _ _ _ _carbs _ _ _ _ _fats _ _ _ _ _proteins

SATURDAY

Macros: _ _ _ _ _carbs _ _ _ _ _fats _ _ _ _ _proteins

SUNDAY

Macros: _ _ _ _ _carbs _ _ _ _ _fats _ _ _ _ _proteins

End of Week Stats

Carbs: __________   Fats: __________   Proteins: __________

Weight: __________   Waist: __________   Hips: __________   Thighs: __________

Arms: __________   Other: __________

Take Inventory

Rate these items on a scale of 1-5, 1 being worst, 5 being best. Add your own if you wish.

Sleep __________   __________   __________

Energy __________   __________   __________

Satiety __________   __________   __________

Mental Clarity __________   __________   __________

Notes

____

____

____

____

____

____

____

____

____

____

____

Notes

Goals

Carbs: _________   Fats: _________   Proteins: _________

Weight: _________   Waist: _________   Hips: _________   Thighs: _________

Arms: _________   Other: _________

Cheat Meal

What Day?   _______________________

What Meal?   _______________________

What Food?   _______________________

Make your cheat meal something indulgent, but still keto-friendly to stay on track! i.e. Keto Ice cream, brownies, etc.

Meal Ideas

____

____

____

____

____

____

____

____

____

____

____

____

<table>
<tr><td>MONDAY</td><td></td></tr>
<tr><td></td><td>Macros: _____carbs _____fats _____proteins</td></tr>
<tr><td>TUESDAY</td><td></td></tr>
<tr><td></td><td>Macros: _____carbs _____fats _____proteins</td></tr>
<tr><td>WEDNESDAY</td><td></td></tr>
<tr><td></td><td>Macros: _____carbs _____fats _____proteins</td></tr>
<tr><td>THURSDAY</td><td></td></tr>
<tr><td></td><td>Macros: _____carbs _____fats _____proteins</td></tr>
<tr><td>FRIDAY</td><td></td></tr>
<tr><td></td><td>Macros: _____carbs _____fats _____proteins</td></tr>
<tr><td>SATURDAY</td><td></td></tr>
<tr><td></td><td>Macros: _____carbs _____fats _____proteins</td></tr>
<tr><td>SUNDAY</td><td></td></tr>
<tr><td></td><td>Macros: _____carbs _____fats _____proteins</td></tr>
</table>

End of Week Stats

Carbs: _________   Fats: _________   Proteins: _________

Weight: _________   Waist: _________   Hips: _________   Thighs: _________

Arms: _________   Other: _________

Take Inventory

Rate these items on a scale of 1-5, 1 being worst, 5 being best. Add your own if you wish.

Sleep _________   _________________   _________

Energy _________   _________________   _________

Satiety _________   _________________   _________

Mental Clarity _________   _________________   _________

Notes

____

____

____

____

____

____

____

____

____

____

Notes

Goals

Carbs: _________   Fats: _________   Proteins: _________

Weight: _________   Waist: _________   Hips: _________   Thighs: _________

Arms: _________   Other: _________

Cheat Meal

What Day? _________________________

What Meal? _________________________

What Food? _________________________

Make your cheat meal something indulgent, but still keto-friendly to stay on track! i.e. Keto Ice cream, brownies, etc.

Meal Ideas

MONDAY

Macros: _____ carbs _____ fats _____ proteins

TUESDAY

Macros: _____ carbs _____ fats _____ proteins

WEDNESDAY

Macros: _____ carbs _____ fats _____ proteins

THURSDAY

Macros: _____ carbs _____ fats _____ proteins

FRIDAY

Macros: _____ carbs _____ fats _____ proteins

SATURDAY

Macros: _____ carbs _____ fats _____ proteins

SUNDAY

Macros: _____ carbs _____ fats _____ proteins

End of Week Stats

Carbs: __________   Fats: __________   Proteins: __________

Weight: __________   Waist: __________   Hips: __________   Thighs: __________

Arms: __________   Other: __________

Take Inventory

Rate these items on a scale of 1-5, 1 being worst, 5 being best. Add your own if you wish.

Sleep __________   __________   __________

Energy __________   __________   __________

Satiety __________   __________   __________

Mental Clarity __________   __________   __________

Notes

____

____

____

____

____

____

____

____

____

____

____

Notes

Goals

Carbs: __________   Fats: __________   Proteins: __________

Weight: __________   Waist: __________   Hips: __________   Thighs: __________

Arms: __________   Other: __________

Cheat Meal

What Day? __________________________

What Meal? __________________________

What Food? __________________________

Make your cheat meal something indulgent, but still keto-friendly to stay on track! i.e. Keto Ice cream, brownies, etc.

Meal Ideas

____

____

____

____

____

____

____

____

____

____

____

<table>
<tr><td>MONDAY</td><td>Macros: _____carbs _____fats _____proteins</td></tr>
<tr><td>TUESDAY</td><td>Macros: _____carbs _____fats _____proteins</td></tr>
<tr><td>WEDNESDAY</td><td>Macros: _____carbs _____fats _____proteins</td></tr>
<tr><td>THURSDAY</td><td>Macros: _____carbs _____fats _____proteins</td></tr>
<tr><td>FRIDAY</td><td>Macros: _____carbs _____fats _____proteins</td></tr>
<tr><td>SATURDAY</td><td>Macros: _____carbs _____fats _____proteins</td></tr>
<tr><td>SUNDAY</td><td>Macros: _____carbs _____fats _____proteins</td></tr>
</table>

End of Week Stats

Carbs: __________   Fats: __________   Proteins: __________

Weight: __________   Waist: __________   Hips: __________   Thighs: __________

Arms: __________   Other: __________

Take Inventory

Rate these items on a scale of 1-5, 1 being worst, 5 being best. Add your own if you wish.

Sleep __________

Energy __________

Satiety __________

Mental Clarity __________

Notes

____

____

____

____

____

____

____

____

____

____

____

____

Notes

Goals

Carbs: ___________   Fats: ___________   Proteins: ___________

Weight: ___________   Waist: ___________   Hips: ___________   Thighs: ___________

Arms: ___________   Other: ___________

Cheat Meal

What Day? _______________________

What Meal? _______________________

What Food? _______________________

Make your cheat meal something indulgent, but still keto-friendly to stay on track! i.e. Keto Ice cream, brownies, etc.

Meal Ideas

____

____

____

____

____

____

____

____

____

____

____

MONDAY

Macros: _____carbs _____fats _____proteins

TUESDAY

Macros: _____carbs _____fats _____proteins

WEDNESDAY

Macros: _____carbs _____fats _____proteins

THURSDAY

Macros: _____carbs _____fats _____proteins

FRIDAY

Macros: _____carbs _____fats _____proteins

SATURDAY

Macros: _____carbs _____fats _____proteins

SUNDAY

Macros: _____carbs _____fats _____proteins

End of Week Stats

Carbs: __________   Fats: __________   Proteins: __________

Weight: __________   Waist: __________   Hips: __________   Thighs: __________

Arms: __________   Other: __________

Take Inventory

Rate these items on a scale of 1-5, 1 being worst, 5 being best. Add your own if you wish.

Sleep __________   __________   __________

Energy __________   __________   __________

Satiety __________   __________   __________

Mental Clarity __________   __________   __________

Notes

____

____

____

____

____

____

____

____

____

____

____

Notes

Goals

Carbs: ___________   Fats: ___________   Proteins: ___________

Weight: ___________   Waist: ___________   Hips: ___________   Thighs: ___________

Arms: ___________   Other: ___________

Cheat Meal

What Day?   ___________________________

What Meal?   ___________________________

What Food?   ___________________________

Make your cheat meal something indulgent, but still keto-friendly to stay on track! i.e. Keto Ice cream, brownies, etc.

Meal Ideas

____

____

____

____

____

____

____

____

____

____

____

MONDAY
Macros: _____carbs _____fats _____proteins

TUESDAY
Macros: _____carbs _____fats _____proteins

WEDNESDAY
Macros: _____carbs _____fats _____proteins

THURSDAY
Macros: _____carbs _____fats _____proteins

FRIDAY
Macros: _____carbs _____fats _____proteins

SATURDAY
Macros: _____carbs _____fats _____proteins

SUNDAY
Macros: _____carbs _____fats _____proteins

End of Week Stats

Carbs: __________   Fats: __________   Proteins: __________

Weight: __________   Waist: __________   Hips: __________   Thighs: __________

Arms: __________   Other: __________

Take Inventory

Rate these items on a scale of 1-5, 1 being worst, 5 being best. Add your own if you wish.

Sleep __________   __________   __________

Energy __________   __________   __________

Satiety __________   __________   __________

Mental Clarity __________   __________   __________

Notes

____

____

____

____

____

____

____

____

____

____

____

Notes

Goals

Carbs: _________   Fats: _________   Proteins: _________

Weight: _________   Waist: _________   Hips: _________   Thighs: _________

Arms: _________   Other: _________

Cheat Meal

What Day?   _______________________________

What Meal?   _______________________________

What Food?   _______________________________

Make your cheat meal something indulgent, but still keto-friendly to stay on track! i.e. Keto Ice cream, brownies, etc.

Meal Ideas

____

____

____

____

____

____

____

____

____

____

____

____

<table>
<tr><td>MONDAY</td><td>Macros: _____carbs _____fats _____proteins</td></tr>
<tr><td>TUESDAY</td><td>Macros: _____carbs _____fats _____proteins</td></tr>
<tr><td>WEDNESDAY</td><td>Macros: _____carbs _____fats _____proteins</td></tr>
<tr><td>THURSDAY</td><td>Macros: _____carbs _____fats _____proteins</td></tr>
<tr><td>FRIDAY</td><td>Macros: _____carbs _____fats _____proteins</td></tr>
<tr><td>SATURDAY</td><td>Macros: _____carbs _____fats _____proteins</td></tr>
<tr><td>SUNDAY</td><td>Macros: _____carbs _____fats _____proteins</td></tr>
</table>

End of Week Stats

Carbs: __________   Fats: __________   Proteins: __________

Weight: __________   Waist: __________   Hips: __________   Thighs: __________

Arms: __________   Other: __________

Take Inventory

Rate these items on a scale of 1-5, 1 being worst, 5 being best. Add your own if you wish.

Sleep __________

Energy __________

Satiety __________

Mental Clarity __________

Notes

____

____

____

____

____

____

____

____

____

____

Notes

Goals

Carbs: _________   Fats: _________   Proteins: _________

Weight: _________   Waist: _________   Hips: _________   Thighs: _________

Arms: _________   Other: _________

Cheat Meal

What Day? _______________________

What Meal? _______________________

What Food? _______________________

Make your cheat meal something indulgent, but still keto-friendly to stay on track! i.e. Keto Ice cream, brownies, etc.

Meal Ideas

____

____

____

____

____

____

____

____

____

____

____

____

<table>
<tr><td>MONDAY</td><td>Macros: _____carbs _____fats _____proteins</td></tr>
<tr><td>TUESDAY</td><td>Macros: _____carbs _____fats _____proteins</td></tr>
<tr><td>WEDNESDAY</td><td>Macros: _____carbs _____fats _____proteins</td></tr>
<tr><td>THURSDAY</td><td>Macros: _____carbs _____fats _____proteins</td></tr>
<tr><td>FRIDAY</td><td>Macros: _____carbs _____fats _____proteins</td></tr>
<tr><td>SATURDAY</td><td>Macros: _____carbs _____fats _____proteins</td></tr>
<tr><td>SUNDAY</td><td>Macros: _____carbs _____fats _____proteins</td></tr>
</table>

End of Week Stats

Carbs: _________   Fats: _________   Proteins: _________

Weight: _________   Waist: _________   Hips: _________   Thighs: _________

Arms: _________   Other: _________

Take Inventory

Rate these items on a scale of 1-5, 1 being worst, 5 being best. Add your own if you wish.

Sleep _________   _________________   _________

Energy _________   _________________   _________

Satiety _________   _________________   _________

Mental Clarity _________   _________________   _________

Notes

____

____

____

____

____

____

____

____

____

____

____

____

Goals

Carbs: _____________   Fats: _____________   Proteins: _____________

Weight: _____________   Waist: _____________   Hips: _____________   Thighs: _____________

Arms: _____________   Other: _____________

Cheat Meal

What Day?   _________________________

What Meal?   _________________________

What Food?   _________________________

Make your cheat meal something indulgent, but still keto-friendly to stay on track! i.e. Keto Ice cream, brownies, etc.

Meal Ideas

____

____

____

____

____

____

____

____

____

____

____

MONDAY

Macros: _____carbs _____fats _____proteins

TUESDAY

Macros: _____carbs _____fats _____proteins

WEDNESDAY

Macros: _____carbs _____fats _____proteins

THURSDAY

Macros: _____carbs _____fats _____proteins

FRIDAY

Macros: _____carbs _____fats _____proteins

SATURDAY

Macros: _____carbs _____fats _____proteins

SUNDAY

Macros: _____carbs _____fats _____proteins

End of Week Stats

Carbs: _____________   Fats: _____________   Proteins: _____________

Weight: _____________   Waist: _____________   Hips: _____________   Thighs: _____________

Arms: _____________   Other: _____________

Take Inventory

Rate these items on a scale of 1-5, 1 being worst, 5 being best. Add your own if you wish.

Sleep   _____________   _____________________________   _____________

Energy   _____________   _____________________________   _____________

Satiety   _____________   _____________________________   _____________

Mental Clarity _____________   _____________________________   _____________

Notes

____

____

____

____

____

____

____

____

____

____

____

Notes

Goals

Carbs: __________   Fats: __________   Proteins: __________

Weight: __________   Waist: __________   Hips: __________   Thighs: __________

Arms: __________   Other: __________

Cheat Meal

What Day?   __________________________

What Meal?   __________________________

What Food?   __________________________

Make your cheat meal something indulgent, but still keto-friendly to stay on track! i.e. Keto Ice cream, brownies, etc.

Meal Ideas

MONDAY
Macros: _____carbs _____fats _____proteins
TUESDAY
Macros: _____carbs _____fats _____proteins
WEDNESDAY
Macros: _____carbs _____fats _____proteins
THURSDAY
Macros: _____carbs _____fats _____proteins
FRIDAY
Macros: _____carbs _____fats _____proteins
SATURDAY
Macros: _____carbs _____fats _____proteins
SUNDAY
Macros: _____carbs _____fats _____proteins

End of Week Stats

Carbs: _________   Fats: _________   Proteins: _________

Weight: _________   Waist: _________   Hips: _________   Thighs: _________

Arms: _________   Other: _________

Take Inventory

Rate these items on a scale of 1–5, 1 being worst, 5 being best. Add your own if you wish.

Sleep _________   _________________   _________

Energy _________   _________________   _________

Satiety _________   _________________   _________

Mental Clarity _________   _________________   _________

Notes

____

____

____

____

____

____

____

____

____

____

Notes

Goals

Carbs: __________   Fats: __________   Proteins: __________

Weight: __________   Waist: __________   Hips: __________   Thighs: __________

Arms: __________   Other: __________

Cheat Meal

What Day? __________________________

What Meal? __________________________

What Food? __________________________

Make your cheat meal something indulgent, but still keto-friendly to stay on track! i.e. Keto Ice cream, brownies, etc.

Meal Ideas

____

____

____

____

____

____

____

____

____

____

____

MONDAY

Macros: _____carbs _____fats _____proteins

TUESDAY

Macros: _____carbs _____fats _____proteins

WEDNESDAY

Macros: _____carbs _____fats _____proteins

THURSDAY

Macros: _____carbs _____fats _____proteins

FRIDAY

Macros: _____carbs _____fats _____proteins

SATURDAY

Macros: _____carbs _____fats _____proteins

SUNDAY

Macros: _____carbs _____fats _____proteins

End of Week Stats

Carbs: __________   Fats: __________   Proteins: __________

Weight: __________   Waist: __________   Hips: __________   Thighs: __________

Arms: __________   Other: __________

Take Inventory

Rate these items on a scale of 1–5, 1 being worst, 5 being best. Add your own if you wish.

Sleep __________

Energy __________

Satiety __________

Mental Clarity __________

Notes

____

____

____

____

____

____

____

____

____

____

Notes

Goals

Carbs: ___________   Fats: ___________   Proteins: ___________

Weight: ___________   Waist: ___________   Hips: ___________   Thighs: ___________

Arms: ___________   Other: ___________

Cheat Meal

What Day? ___________________________

What Meal? ___________________________

What Food? ___________________________

Make your cheat meal something indulgent, but still keto-friendly to stay on track! i.e. Keto Ice cream, brownies, etc.

Meal Ideas

____

____

____

____

____

____

____

____

____

____

____

<table>
<tr><td>MONDAY</td><td>Macros: _____carbs _____fats _____proteins</td></tr>
<tr><td>TUESDAY</td><td>Macros: _____carbs _____fats _____proteins</td></tr>
<tr><td>WEDNESDAY</td><td>Macros: _____carbs _____fats _____proteins</td></tr>
<tr><td>THURSDAY</td><td>Macros: _____carbs _____fats _____proteins</td></tr>
<tr><td>FRIDAY</td><td>Macros: _____carbs _____fats _____proteins</td></tr>
<tr><td>SATURDAY</td><td>Macros: _____carbs _____fats _____proteins</td></tr>
<tr><td>SUNDAY</td><td>Macros: _____carbs _____fats _____proteins</td></tr>
</table>

End of Week Stats

Carbs: __________   Fats: __________   Proteins: __________

Weight: __________   Waist: __________   Hips: __________   Thighs: __________

Arms: __________   Other: __________

Take Inventory

Rate these items on a scale of 1-5, 1 being worst, 5 being best. Add your own if you wish.

Sleep __________

Energy __________

Satiety __________

Mental Clarity __________

Notes

____

____

____

____

____

____

____

____

____

____

Notes

Goals

Carbs: __________   Fats: __________   Proteins: __________

Weight: __________   Waist: __________   Hips: __________   Thighs: __________

Arms: __________   Other: __________

Cheat Meal

What Day? __________________________

What Meal? __________________________

What Food? __________________________

Make your cheat meal something indulgent, but still keto-friendly to stay on track! i.e. Keto Ice cream, brownies, etc.

Meal Ideas

MONDAY	Macros: _____carbs _____fats _____proteins
TUESDAY	Macros: _____carbs _____fats _____proteins
WEDNESDAY	Macros: _____carbs _____fats _____proteins
THURSDAY	Macros: _____carbs _____fats _____proteins
FRIDAY	Macros: _____carbs _____fats _____proteins
SATURDAY	Macros: _____carbs _____fats _____proteins
SUNDAY	Macros: _____carbs _____fats _____proteins

End of Week Stats

Carbs: __________   Fats: __________   Proteins: __________

Weight: __________   Waist: __________   Hips: __________   Thighs: __________

Arms: __________   Other: __________

Take Inventory

Rate these items on a scale of 1-5, 1 being worst, 5 being best. Add your own if you wish.

Sleep __________

Energy __________

Satiety __________

Mental Clarity __________

Notes

____

____

____

____

____

____

____

____

____

____

____

Notes

Goals

Carbs: ___________   Fats: ___________   Proteins: ___________

Weight: ___________   Waist: ___________   Hips: ___________   Thighs: ___________

Arms: ___________   Other: ___________

Cheat Meal

What Day? _________________________

What Meal? _________________________

What Food? _________________________

Make your cheat meal something indulgent, but still keto-friendly to stay on track! i.e. Keto Ice cream, brownies, etc.

Meal Ideas

____

____

____

____

____

____

____

____

____

____

____

____

MONDAY

Macros: _ _ _ _ _carbs _ _ _ _ _fats _ _ _ _ _proteins

TUESDAY

Macros: _ _ _ _ _carbs _ _ _ _ _fats _ _ _ _ _proteins

WEDNESDAY

Macros: _ _ _ _ _carbs _ _ _ _ _fats _ _ _ _ _proteins

THURSDAY

Macros: _ _ _ _ _carbs _ _ _ _ _fats _ _ _ _ _proteins

FRIDAY

Macros: _ _ _ _ _carbs _ _ _ _ _fats _ _ _ _ _proteins

SATURDAY

Macros: _ _ _ _ _carbs _ _ _ _ _fats _ _ _ _ _proteins

SUNDAY

Macros: _ _ _ _ _carbs _ _ _ _ _fats _ _ _ _ _proteins

End of Week Stats

Carbs: _________   Fats: _________   Proteins: _________

Weight: _________   Waist: _________   Hips: _________   Thighs: _________

Arms: _________   Other: _________

Take Inventory

Rate these items on a scale of 1-5, 1 being worst, 5 being best. Add your own if you wish.

Sleep _________

Energy _________

Satiety _________

Mental Clarity _________

Notes

____

____

____

____

____

____

____

____

____

____

Notes

Notes

Goals

Carbs: _________   Fats: _________   Proteins: _________

Weight: _________   Waist: _________   Hips: _________   Thighs: _________

Arms: _________   Other: _________

Cheat Meal

What Day?   _______________________

What Meal?   _______________________

What Food?   _______________________

Make your cheat meal something indulgent, but still keto-friendly to stay on track! i.e. Keto Ice cream, brownies, etc.

Meal Ideas

____

____

____

____

____

____

____

____

____

____

____

MONDAY	
	Macros: _____carbs _____fats _____proteins

TUESDAY	
	Macros: _____carbs _____fats _____proteins

WEDNESDAY	
	Macros: _____carbs _____fats _____proteins

THURSDAY	
	Macros: _____carbs _____fats _____proteins

FRIDAY	
	Macros: _____carbs _____fats _____proteins

SATURDAY	
	Macros: _____carbs _____fats _____proteins

SUNDAY	
	Macros: _____carbs _____fats _____proteins

End of Week Stats

Carbs: __________   Fats: __________   Proteins: __________

Weight: __________   Waist: __________   Hips: __________   Thighs: __________

Arms: __________   Other: __________

Take Inventory

Rate these items on a scale of 1-5, 1 being worst, 5 being best. Add your own if you wish.

Sleep   __________   __________________   __________

Energy   __________   __________________   __________

Satiety   __________   __________________   __________

Mental Clarity   __________   __________________   __________

Notes

____

____

____

____

____

____

____

____

____

____

Notes